THE
CONSCIENTIOUS
VISITOR

25 Ways to Really Help
When Someone You Love
is Ill or Dying

Azalea Art Press

Southern Pines, North Carolina

ISBN: 978-0-9899961-1-2

ACKNOWLEDGMENTS

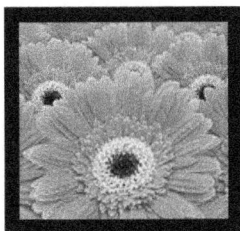

We wish to thank the nurses and
staff at Sunrise Assisted Living
and Vitas Innovative Hospice Care
in Oakland, California
for their valuable advice.

Our gratitude also goes to
The Roeper Family—Tom, Peter and
Karen—who offered many good ideas
and helpful support.

Most of all we want to thank
Dr. Annemarie Roeper
(1918-2012)
who was the inspiration
for this book.

All healing is first
a healing of the heart.

- Carl Townsend

Dear Friends:

Over the past 25 years, we have had many experiences being close to those who were seriously ill or who were dying.

This book provides some practical thoughts for giving support to family, doctors, nurses, caregivers and to the patients themselves.

May these ideas inspire all of us to provide the highest possible level of care for our loved ones.

Respectfully,

Marla Lay
Karen Mireau

November 2013

INTRODUCTION

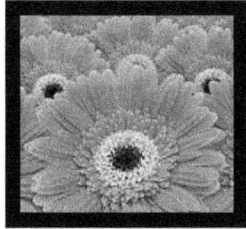

We all want to be helpful to our friends and loved ones when they are in a medical crisis. However, at times our actions, no matter how well-intended, may be counterproductive to a patient's care and overall well being.

We believe that being a good visitor or caregiver to those who are ill is a skill that can be easily learned. This guide provides clear, practical advice for making a patient's experience better as well as specific ways to lend support to family and caregivers.

There is so much more to being ill than we can sometimes imagine. If someone you love is seriously or chronically ill, it's difficult to know exactly how the sick person feels.

We often don't know what to do or what to say that might be really helpful to the patient. Being a visitor in a hospital or hospice setting is uncomfortable for most people and this further amplifies the emotions and feelings we have when someone we love is in crisis.

Even the simplest acts can be very meaningful to someone who is ill. A card or a short phone call from you can do wonders. The important thing is to make contact and to express caring. Perhaps the best general advice is to keep visits short, calm and quiet —unless, of course, your patient is in a celebratory mood!

Remember that caregivers are people who devote their positive energy to healing others and that they really care deeply about their patients. They are there to help you, too, and their advice can be invaluable.

THE
CONSCIENTIOUS
VISITOR

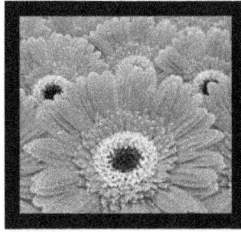

1.
Tell the truth.
Fear of illness and death is something we all
share, but honesty is almost always preferable
to sugarcoating a serious situation. Be direct
with the patient about their prognosis—
always tempered with sensitivity,
understanding and good discretion.

2.
Stay hopeful.
Maintain a sense of hopefulness. Even
terminal patients should be seen beyond their
illness and treated like whole human beings
with a future, no matter how short
or long their time with us may be.

3.
Listen with the heart.
Be a good listener. Our human need to share
our story does not diminish during an illness.
Silence is sometimes necessary, too.

3.
(Cont.)
Just being present physically often provides great comfort. Assure your loved one that all conversations will be kept confidential.

4.
Speak from the heart.
Be gently stimulating by asking questions and encouraging positive conversation. Don't be afraid to talk about death or difficult subjects.

5.
Treat patients respectfully.
Talk with the patient like any good friend— sit at eye-level and speak to them directly. Ask them what they need or want that may be overlooked by others.

6.
Give advice with sensitivity to caregivers.
Know that the average caregiver gives a great deal of themselves to the care of their patient. Be slow to criticize. Remember: there is a lot going on behind the scenes that you may not know about. Ask questions and collect more information about your specific concerns

6.

(Cont.)

It may be that what you would like done is already in motion or is against medical advice. Ask the caregiver what you could do to be helpful. Then, if something more or different can be done, everyone can feel good about it

7.

Stay neutral.

Refrain from getting involved in family disputes or politics. Be supportive to everyone by staying neutral and focusing on the patient's needs.

8.

Keep visit times respectful.

Allow the patient to have proper rest by being sensitive to their energy levels. Respect hospital rules and schedule visit times that are convenient for all concerned—including the patient, family, caregivers, nurses and doctors. Keep visits short. Plan them for when the patient really needs or wants company. Too many visitors at one time can be overwhelming for the patient.

9.
Visit when you are healthy.
People who are ill often have very weak
immune systems. If you have a cold or flu,
schedule an alternate visit time. Remember
to wash your hands before—and after—
your visit.

10.
Encourage independence.
Some people are sensitive to feeling like an
invalid. Unless requested by the patient or
required by their doctor, refrain from doing
things that patients can do for themselves—
it will help the person who is ill feel they are
still competent. However, do insure that the
person who is sick has their true needs met.
Use your intuition and best judgment on how
helpful (or not) to be at any moment.

11.
Minister only with permission.
Offer religious or spiritual support only
if the patient wants and agrees to it.
Avoid evangelizing or promoting your own
religion or philosophy, especially if it conflicts
with the patient's own beliefs.

12.
Be tolerant of erratic patient behavior.
Illness can often cause a sudden change in a patient's personality, especially after a stroke. Remember that the patient may be struggling with both physical and emotional issues at once, and may not be their best selves.

13.
Ask for help.
It's natural to want to help our loved ones as much as possible, but it's difficult to be effective when you are stressed or over-whelmed. If you are a primary caregiver, don't be afraid to ask for help from family or friends.

14.
Take care of caregivers.
Supporters need a lot of support. Periodically ask the family members or caregivers if they would like an hour of free time so that they can take a walk or do an errand. Offer to sit and talk with the patient, read a book to them, or just be there with them in their room. Even a short break can be helpful and reduce stress for everyone.

15.
Share a pet.
Animal love can be very healing and cheering.
With permission, bring a snuggly,
well-behaved pet for a short visit.

16.
Be a health nut.
Nutrition is important, especially for those
who are ill. Dietary requirements often change
from day to day. Find out what kinds of
healthful foods the patient likes (and the
doctor recommends) and offer to bring these
instead of candy or sweets.

17.
Be a household angel.
Ask if you can take care of pets, plants, mail,
laundry, dry cleaning, or anything in the
patient's household that could use attention
or a watchful eye.

18.
Use a soft touch.
Human contact is very important to healing,
but people often shy away from touching
others who are sick.

18.
(Cont.)

If you are comfortable, ask the patient if they would like a hug or a very gentle foot or hand massage. Also, offer to help with personal grooming, which sometimes is given less attention during an illness.

19.
Be a nurturing friend.

Relate to the person as you always have. Talk about the things you have always talked about. It will give the person a renewed feeling of normalcy. Reassure them that they are not their illness and that you are still their friend.

20.
Offer a change of scenery.

Ask if you can accompany the patient on a walk if they are able, or take them for ride in their wheelchair. Fresh air and sunshine or even a brief change of atmosphere can do a world of good.

21.
Help maintain schedules.
Offer to help maintain the patient's physical therapy, medication or nutritional plan, when appropriate. Another helpful role would be to handle inquiries and update others on the patient's condition so that family can focus on the patient's immediate needs.

22.
Practice compassion for all.
Your loved one's illness can be an opportunity to practice love and compassion towards the patient and others, but don't forget yourself. To be most effective, rest, eat well and take care of your own health during this time.

23.
Plan ahead.
If you are the family or primary caregiver, try to be prepared for possible health situations by investigating hospice or palliative care before it becomes necessary. They offer a wide range of services that are often free or low cost and can help you prepare and plan wisely for the days ahead.

24.

Be a love bug.

Reassure the patient and their family that they are well loved and cared for on a regular basis. This may be the best medicine of all!

25.

Know you are loved, too.

Even the smallest of your loving, caring and thoughtful actions will not go unnoticed by the patient or those around you.
Your presence may be one of the most important gifts you can possibly give your friend or loved one.

RESACERS

RESOURCES

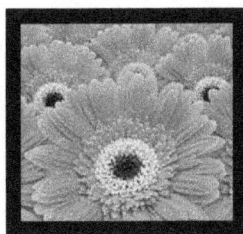

Resources
Books

Dying Well
Ira Byock, M.D.
Riverhead Books / Berkley publishing Group, 1997.
Comprehensive book about death with dignity.

The End of Life Handbook
David B. Feldman, PH.D.
S. Andrew Lasher, Jr., M.D.
New Harbinger Publications, Inc., 2007.
Covers all aspects of the medical, physical, social and emotional aspects of caring for a loved one.

Final Gifts
Maggie Callanan and Patricia Kelley
Bantam Books, 1992.
Christian view on spirituality near death.

The Four Things That Matter Most
Ira Byock, M.D.
Free Press / Simon & Schuster, Inc., 2004.
True stories of healing relationships at the end of life.

The Grief Recovery Handbook
Russell Friedman
HarperCollins, 2009.
Clear advice for families who are grieving.

**Guide to Caregiving
in the Final Months of Life**
Betsy Murphy, RN, FNP, CHPN
TM Brown Publishers, Inc., 2007.
http://www.GuidetoCaregiving.com
*Advice from a hospice nurse on caregiving during the
process of dying.*

Handbook for Mortals
Joanne Lynn, M.D. and Joan Harrold, M.D.
Oxford University Press, 1999.
*Straight-forward instruction manual for patients with
serious or terminal illness.*

**How to be a Friend
to a Friend Who's Sick**
Lotty Cottin Pogrebin
PublicAffairs, 2013.
*A comprehensive guidebook for relating in more
meaningful ways to friends or family who are ill.*

The Needs of the Dying
David Kessler
Quill / HarperCollins, 2001.
Guide to treating those who are ill or dying as whole human beings.

Passages in Caregiving:
Turning Chaos into Confidence
Gail Sheehy
Harper Paperback, 2011.
Solid, practical advice by the author of Passages.

On Grief and Grieving
Elisabeth Kubler-Ross and David Kessler
Scribner, 2005.
A full exploration of the stages of grieving, which dispels the myth that everyone experiences grief in the same way.

Resources
Online

We recommend searching topics such as "how to comfort a sick friend" or "talking with a sick person" to find the most current articles and forums.

www.americanhospice.org
American Hospice Foundation

www.caringbridge.org
Excellent online tool for communication between friends and family of the patient

www.death-and-dying.org
Buddhist inspiration

http://dying.about.com/b/2010/11/08/
hospice-care-vs-palliative-care.html
Good description of hospice -vs- palliative care

http://grief.com
The work of grief experts David Kessler & Elisabeth Kubler-Ross

www.goodgrief.org
Hindu inspiration

www.griefnet.org
Informational site

www.hellogrief.org
Articles on grieving

http://hospicefoundation.org
Hospice Foundation of America

http://topics.nytimes.com/
top/news/health/
diseasesconditionshealthtopics/
deathanddying/index.html
Articles and resources on death and dying

www.pbs.org/wnet
onourownterms
Bill Moyers on dying

Resources
Periodicals

Five Wishes / Aging With Dignity (www.agingwithdignity.org/five-wishes. php) A patient care booklet that provides a way to discuss and decide all issues surrounding end-of-life care. Once filled out and signed, it is legally valid in most states.

ABOUT THE AUTHORS

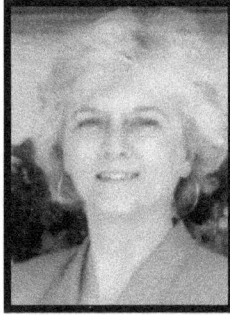

Marla Lay has been a caregiver and counselor for over thirty years. She is currently a health researcher and assists others in evaluating alternative medical treatments and options.

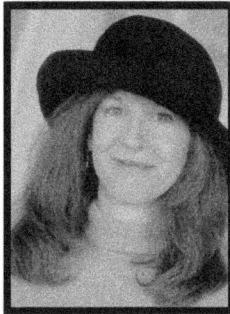

Karen Mireau is founder of Azalea Art Press. She has enjoyed writing about health, healing and spirituality for the last three decades.

Notes:

Azalea Art Press
specializes in giving personal attention
to authors who wish to realize
their literary and creative dreams.

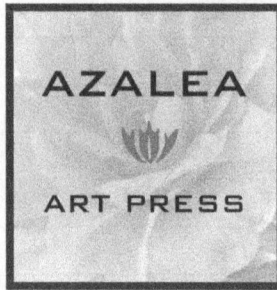

AZALEA

ART PRESS

To learn more about writing,
designing and successfully marketing
your next print, e-reader or e-book,
please get in touch with:

Karen Mireau
Azalea.Art.Press@gmail.com
azaleaartpress.blogspot.com

www.ingramcontent.com/pod-product-compliance
Lightning Source LLC
Chambersburg PA
CBHW021123020426
42331CB00004B/602